Made in the USA
Middletown, DE
09 March 2023

26461059R00068